Chronic Fatigue Diet Cookbook:

Easy and Delicious Recipes for People with Chronic Fatigue Syndrome

Andrew J. Nettles

Disclaimer

Copyright © 2023 by Andrew J. Nettles

The information provided in this book is for general informational purposes only. The author and publisher of this book have made every effort to ensure the accuracy and completeness of the content. However, they do not guarantee or warrant the information's reliability, applicability, or suitability for any specific individual or purpose.

The content of this book is based on the author's research, personal experiences, and opinions. It is not intended to replace or substitute for professional medical, dietary, or fitness advice. Readers should consult with qualified healthcare professionals or certified experts before changing their diet, exercise routine, or lifestyle.

By reading this book, you acknowledge that you have read and understood this disclaimer and agree to hold harmless the author, publisher, and any associated parties from any liability or damages arising from using this book.

Table of Content

Introduction

Energy levels may be increased, inflammation can be reduced, and the immune system can be strengthened with a balanced diet.

Eating a wide range of fruits, veggies, healthy grains, and lean meats is important. Staying hydrated and avoiding prepared foods, sugary drinks, and too much coffee is also significant.

Chronic fatigue syndrome (CFS) can be seen as a complicated disorder that brings about a variety of symptoms, including weariness, cognitive issues, muscular pain, and sleep abnormalities. Eating a healthy diet are things that people can do to manage their symptoms.

This cookbook provides easy and delicious recipes perfect for people with CFS. The recipes are all made with whole, unprocessed ingredients and are designed to be both nutritious and flavorful. Whether looking for a quick breakfast, a light lunch, or a hearty dinner, you will find something you like in this book.

In addition to the recipes, this cookbook also includes information about the role of diet in managing CFS and tips for cooking and eating when you are tired. Following the advice in this book can improve your overall health and well-being and manage your CFS symptoms more effectively.

What is Chronic Fatigue Syndrome (CFS)

Chronic fatigue syndrome (CFS), or myalgic encephalomyelitis (ME), is a long-term ailment that causes extreme fatigue that does not go away with rest. People with CFS may also have other symptoms, such as muscle pain, cognitive problems, and sleep disturbances.

Although the cause of CFS is unclear, researchers believe several variables, including infections, genetics, and environmental triggers, are likely responsible. Although there is no known therapy for CFS, there are ways to manage the symptoms.

CFS can have a significant impact on a person's life. Working, attending school, or participating in social activities can make it difficult. Additionally, it may result in issues with depression, anxiety, and other mental health issues.

If you think you may have CFS, it is important to see a doctor. No one test can diagnose CFS, but your specialist can rule out other conditions that may be causing your symptoms.

There is no one-size-fits-all treatment for CFS, but several things can help manage the symptoms. These include:

Getting regular exercise, even if it is just for short periods, Eating a healthy diet, Getting enough sleep, Managing stress, Avoiding caffeine and alcohol,

Getting Support From Friends And Family

If you have CFS, it is important to remember that you are not alone. Many people are living with this condition. Resources are also accessible to help you properly manage your symptoms and live a full life.

The Role of Diet in Managing CFS

No one-size-fits-all diet exists for people with chronic fatigue syndrome (CFS). Still, some general dietary guidelines can help to improve energy levels, reduce inflammation, and boost the immune system.

Consume lots of veggies and fruit: Fruits and vegetables are packed with vitamins, minerals, and antioxidants that can help to improve overall health and well-being. They are a healthy option for those wanting to reduce or maintain a healthy weight because they are low in calories and fat.

Select whole grains instead of processed ones: Fiber-rich foods like whole grains might help you feel full and satisfied longer. Additionally, they are a wonderful source of B vitamins, which are crucial for generating energy.

Include lean protein in your diet: Lean protein, such as chicken, fish, beans, and tofu, can help to build and repair muscle tissue.

Limit processed food: Processed meals are generally substantial in calories, sugar, and unhealthy fats. They can also be low in nutrients. It is best to limit your intake of processed foods and focus on eating whole, unprocessed foods.

Stay hydrated: It is important to stay hydrated, especially if you are experiencing fatigue. Drink plenty of water, unsweetened tea, or sparkling water throughout the day.

Avoid caffeine and alcohol: Caffeine and alcohol can both dehydrate you and make fatigue worse. Best to avoid them if you have CFS.

Listen to your body: Eating when you are hungry and resting when you are tired is vital. Don't push yourself too hard, as this can worsen your symptoms.

If you have CFS, you must talk to your doctor about how to manage your symptoms. They can help you create a personalized diet plan for you.

Nutritional Guidelines for CFS

There are no specific nutritional guidelines for people with chronic fatigue syndrome (CFS), but some general dietary recommendations may be helpful. These include:

- Eating a balanced diet includes plenty of fruits, vegetables, and whole grains.
- Getting enough protein.
- Limiting processed foods, sugary drinks, and excessive caffeine.
- Staying hydrated.
- Listening to your body, eating when you are hungry, and resting when you are tired.

It is also important to talk to your doctor about any dietary changes you are considering, as they can help you create a personalized plan that is right for you.

Specific Foods For People With CFS

Fruits and veggies: These foods are full of vitamins, minerals, and chemicals that can help improve your health and well-being. They also have few calories and fat, making them a decent choice for people who want to lose weight or keep it healthy.

Whole grains: Another excellent source of fiber is whole grains, which, among other benefits, may help you feel fuller for longer. They are also a good source of B vitamins, which are important for energy production.

Lean protein: Lean protein, such as chicken, fish, beans, and tofu, can help to build and repair muscle tissue.

It's also a good source of iron, which is essential for red blood cell production.

Healthy fats: Healthy fats, including those in nuts, seeds, and olive oil, may aid in reducing inflammation and promoting heart health.

Fermented foods: Yogurt, sauerkraut, and kimchi are examples of fermented foods that are high in probiotics, a kind of helpful bacteria that may enhance gut health.

Water: It is important to stay hydrated, especially if you are experiencing fatigue. Drink plenty of water, unsweetened tea, or sparkling water throughout the day.

It is also important to avoid certain foods that may worsen CFS symptoms. These include:

Processed foods: Processed foods are often high in calories, sugar, and unhealthy fats. They can also be low in nutrients.

Sugary drinks: Sugary drinks can lead to weight gain and inflammation, both of which can worsen CFS symptoms.

Caffeine: Caffeine can dehydrate you and make fatigue worse.

Alcohol: Alcohol can dehydrate you and make fatigue worse. If you have CFS, you must talk to your doctor about how to manage your symptoms. They can help you create a personalized diet plan for you.

Tips for Cooking and Eating When You're Tired

Finding the energy to cook a healthy meal can be hard if you're tired. But eating nutritious foods is important for staying healthy and managing fatigue. Here are some tips for cooking and eating when you're tired:

Plan: It is advisable to plan your meals for the coming week during the weekend. When you're exhausted throughout the week, this will help you save time and effort.

Make meals easy to prepare: Many recipes are available for quick and easy meals. Look for recipes that call for simple ingredients and don't require much cooking time.

Use convenience foods: There's no shame in using convenience foods when you're short on time or energy. Frozen vegetables, canned beans, and pre-cooked chicken are healthy and convenient options.

Get help from others: If you have family or friends willing to help, ask them to cook or help you with meal prep.

Don't be afraid to eat out: Eating out is a perfectly acceptable option if you don't have the energy to cook. Just be sure to choose healthy options when you eat out.

Listen to your body: Don't push yourself if you're too tired to cook. It's okay to order takeout or eat a simple meal. The most important thing is to eat something that will give you the energy you need to get through the day.

Here are some additional tips for cooking and eating when you're tired:

Set realistic expectations. Don't try to cook a gourmet meal when you're tired. Instead, focus on making something simple and nutritious.

Don't be afraid to experiment. There are many different ways to cook healthy meals.

Make cooking fun. If you enjoy cooking, it will be less of a chore when you're tired. Put on some music and make it a relaxing experience.

Recipes For People With CFS

Breakfast

Oatmeal with Blueberries and Almonds

Ingredients:

1 cup rolled oats

2 cups water

1/2 cup blueberries

1/4 cup sliced almonds

One teaspoon of ground cinnamon

1/2 teaspoon maple syrup (optional)

Instructions:

In a medium pan, bring the water to a boil.

The pot should now include oats, blueberries, almonds, and cinnamon.

Stirring periodically, lower the heat to low and simmer for five minutes.

If using maple syrup, take the oats off the heat and mix it in.

Serve right away.

Tips:

Add milk or yogurt to the saucepan before stirring the oats for creamier oatmeal.

Add other fruits, nuts, or seeds to your oatmeal. Some popular additions include bananas, strawberries, walnuts, and chia seeds.

If you are short on time, you can make overnight oats. Combine the oats, milk, yogurt, and other desired ingredients in a jar or container. Cover and refrigerate overnight. In the morning, your oatmeal will be ready to eat!

Yogurt Parfait with Fruit and Granola

Ingredients:

1 cup plain yogurt

1/2 cup granola

1/2 cup fresh fruit (such as berries, sliced bananas, or chopped nuts)

Honey or maple syrup (optional)

Instructions:

Layer the yogurt, granola, and fruit in a glass or container.

Up till the top of the glass or jar, keep adding layers.

If desired, drizzle with honey or maple syrup.

Either serve right now or store in the fridge.

Tips:

You can use cereal, oats, or even cookies if you don't have granola.

Get creative with your fruit choices. There are endless possibilities!

You can add other toppings to your parfait, such as nuts, seeds, or chocolate chips.

Eggs Benedict with Spinach and Asparagus

Ingredients:

6 English muffins, split and toasted

12 slices Canadian bacon

Six eggs

1 cup water

1/4 cup white vinegar

1/4 cup (1/2 stick) unsalted butter

1/4 teaspoon salt

1/4 teaspoon ground black pepper

1/2 cup chopped fresh spinach

1/2 cup cooked asparagus, cut into 1-inch pieces

Instructions:

Put the vinegar in a big pot of water and heat it over medium heat until it bubbles.

Each egg should be cracked into a small bowl.

Slide the eggs carefully into the water that is already boiling.

Cook for 3–4 mins until the whites are set, but the yolks are still runny.

Make the hollandaise sauce while the eggs are cooking.

In a small saucepan over low heat, melt the butter.

Whisk the egg whites, salt, and pepper in a small bowl.

Stir the melted butter into the egg yolk mixture slowly with a whisk. Whisk the sauce until it gets thick and smooth.

Put a slice of Canadian bacon on each half of an English muffin to make the Eggs Benedict. Add a cooked egg, spinach, and asparagus to the top. Serve right away. Drizzle with Hollandaise sauce.

Tips:

To ensure your poached eggs are cooked properly, use a slotted spoon to slowly stir the water in a circular motion before adding the eggs. This will cause a swirl that will help the eggs cook evenly.

You can also make the hollandaise sauce and warm it gently before serving.

Eggs Benedict is a popular meal dish that can also be eaten for breakfast, lunch, or dinner.

Lunch

Salad with Grilled Chicken or Fish

Ingredients:

One head of romaine lettuce, washed and chopped

1/2 cup chopped cucumber

1/2 cup chopped tomato

1/4 cup chopped red onion

1/4 cup chopped green bell pepper

1/4 cup crumbled feta cheese

1/4 cup olive oil

Two tablespoons of red wine vinegar

One teaspoon of Dijon mustard

1/2 teaspoon salt

1/4 teaspoon black pepper

1/2 cup grilled chicken or fish, shredded

Instructions:

Combine the lettuce, cucumber, tomato, red onion, green bell pepper, and feta cheese in a large bowl.

In a small bowl, Olive oil should be mixed with red wine vinegar, Dijon mustard, salt, and black pepper.

Toss the salad with the dressing after spreading it.

Top with the grilled chicken or fish and serve immediately.

Tips:

You can use any lettuce you like. Romaine is a good choice because it has a sturdy texture that can hold up to the dressing and toppings.

If you don't have feta cheese, you can use any cheese you like. Cheddar, Parmesan, or goat cheese would all be good choices.

Add other toppings to your salad, such as croutons, avocado, or hard-boiled eggs.

Salads are a great way to get your daily fruits, vegetables, and protein dose. Grilled chicken or fish is a healthy and delicious way to add protein to your salad.

Soup and Sandwich

Soup and sandwich is a classic lunch combination that is both delicious and satisfying. There are many different types of soup and sandwich combinations that you can try, so you can find one that suits your taste.

Here are a few ideas for soup Ideas and sandwich combinations:

- Tomato soup and grilled cheese sandwich
- Chicken noodle soup and a club sandwich
- French onion soup and a grilled ham and cheese sandwich
- Clam chowder and a BLT sandwich
- Minestrone soup and a turkey sandwich

You can also get creative with your soup and sandwich combinations. For example, try a grilled cheese sandwich with tomato soup or a turkey sandwich with cranberry sauce.

You will surely enjoy a delicious and satisfying meal no matter what type of soup and sandwich combination you choose.

Tips for making a great soup and sandwich:

- Use fresh ingredients whenever possible.
- Make sure the soup is hot, and the sandwich is toasted.
- Use a variety of toppings to add flavor and interest to your sandwich.
- Serve your soup and sandwich with your favorite chips or salad.

Dinner

Chicken Stir-Fry with Vegetables

Ingredients:

1-pound boneless, skinless chicken breast cut into 1-inch chunks.

One tablespoon cornstarch

One teaspoon salt

1/2 teaspoon black pepper

One tablespoon of vegetable oil

One onion, chopped

Two cloves garlic, minced

One red bell pepper, chopped

One green bell pepper, chopped

1 cup broccoli florets

1/2 cup snow peas

1/4 cup soy sauce

1/4 cup chicken broth

One tablespoon honey

One teaspoon of sesame oil

Instructions:

Combine the chicken, cornstarch, salt, and pepper in a medium bowl. Toss to coat.

Vegetable oil should be heated in a large pan or wok over medium-high heat.

Add the chicken and simmer it thoroughly while stirring periodically.

The chicken should be taken out of the pan and put aside.

Stirring regularly, add the onion and garlic to the pan, and simmer until tender.

When the veggies are tender-crisp, add the broccoli, snow peas, red and green bell peppers, and simmer, stirring periodically.

Add the soy sauce, broth, honey, and sesame oil to the pan with the chicken once more.

When the mixture boils, turn down the heat, cover, and simmer for five minutes or until the sauce has thickened.

Serve immediately over rice or noodles.

Tips:

In your stir-fry, you may use whatever veggies you desire. Carrots, mushrooms, zucchini, and water chestnuts are common options.

If you don't have any chicken, you may substitute tofu or shrimp in your stir-fry.

Add extras to your stir-fry, such as rice, noodles, or eggs.

Stir-fries are a fast and simple method to prepare a tasty and nutritious supper.

Salmon with Roasted Potatoes and Green Beans

Ingredients:

1 pound salmon fillets, skin on or off

One tablespoon of olive oil

One teaspoon salt

1/2 teaspoon black pepper

1 pound small red potatoes, quartered

1 pound green beans, trimmed

1/4 cup balsamic vinegar

1/4 cup honey

One tablespoon of Dijon mustard

Instructions:

Preheat oven to (200 degrees C).

Toss the salmon, olive oil, salt, and pepper in a large bowl.

On a baking sheet covered with parchment paper, put the salmon.

Toss the potatoes, green beans, balsamic vinegar, honey, and Dijon mustard in a separate bowl.

Spread the vegetables around the salmon on the baking sheet.

Bake for 20-25 mins until the salmon is cooked and the vegetables are tender.

Serve immediately.

Tips:

You can also use any potatoes you like in this recipe. Yukon Gold, red, or sweet potatoes would all be good choices.

If you don't have balsamic vinegar, use any vinegar you like.

Red wine vinegar or white wine vinegar would both be good choices.

Some popular choices include garlic powder, onion powder, and Italian seasoning.

Salmon with roasted potatoes and green beans is a healthy and delicious meal for a weeknight dinner.

Spaghetti with Meat Sauce

Ingredients:

1 pound ground beef

One onion, chopped

Two cloves garlic, minced

1 (28-ounce) can of crushed tomatoes

1 (15-ounce) can of tomato sauce

1 (15-ounce) can of tomato paste

One teaspoon of dried oregano

One teaspoon of dried basil

One teaspoon salt

1/2 teaspoon black pepper

12 ounces spaghetti

Parmesan cheese, for garnish

Instructions:

Brown the ground beef, onion, and garlic on medium heat in a big saucepan. Get rid of any extra fat.

Add the oregano, basil, tomato paste, crushed tomatoes, tomato sauce, salt, and pepper. Until the sauce has thickened, simmer for an hour on low heat after bringing it to a simmer.

Meanwhile, prepare the spaghetti as directed on the package.

To serve, divide the spaghetti among bowls and top with the meat sauce. Garnish with Parmesan cheese and serve immediately.

Spaghetti with meat sauce is a classic Italian dish for family dinners. It is also a great way to use up leftover ground beef.

Snacks

Combine your favorite nuts, seeds, dried fruit, and chocolate chips in a jar or bag.

Hard-boiled eggs are a convenient and healthful snack that can be cooked beforehand.

Carefully place eggs in a pot of cold water and bring to a boil. Cover the pot and remove the water from the heat once the water is boiling.

Allow the eggs to sit in the hot water for 12 mins, then drain and rinse with cold water.

Yogurt parfaits are delicious and nutritious snacks that can be made in minutes. Layer yogurt, fruit, granola, and nuts in a glass or jar.

Snacks made of fruits and vegetables are a terrific way to achieve your recommended daily intake of these foods. Wash and chop your favorite fruits and vegetables and enjoy.

Cheese and crackers are a classic snack that is always a hit. Pair your favorite cheese with crackers or bread.

Popcorn is a light and nutritious snack that may be prepared in the microwave or stovetop. Pop your popcorn and enjoy.

Frozen grapes are a good and healthy snack for a hot day. Wash and freeze grapes, then enjoy.

Trail mix bars are an excellent way to enjoy trail mix on the go. Combine your favorite trail mix ingredients in a food processor and pulse until well combined.

The mixture should be pressed into a baking dish, then refrigerated for at least 30 minutes before being cut into bars.

Energy bites are a healthy and delicious snack perfect for a pre-workout or quick pick-me-up. Combine your favorite nut butter, oats, honey, and chocolate chips in a food processor and pulse until well combined. Roll the mixture into balls and enjoy.

Dried fruit is a healthy and portable snack that can be made ahead of time. Wash and slice your favorite fruits and place them in a dehydrator or oven set to the lowest setting. Dehydrate the fruit for 6-8 hours until it is dry and leathery.

Nuts are a nutritious and satisfying treat that may be had on their own or in soups, trail mixes, and yogurt.

Seeds are a healthy and nutritious snack high in protein and fiber. Some popular seeds include chia seeds, flax seeds, and pumpkin seeds.

Dark chocolate is a healthy and delicious snack that is high in antioxidants. Choose a dark chocolate bar with at least 70% cocoa content.

Fruit

Fruits are a great way to get fiber, vitamins, and minerals. You can eat them raw, cook them, or make juice from them. Here are some fruit recipes and tips on how to prepare them:

Fresh fruit

Wash all fruit thoroughly before eating.

Cut fruit into bite-sized pieces or slices.

Serve fruit with a variety of dips, such as yogurt, hummus, or guacamole.

Add fruit to salads, cereal, or yogurt.

Make fruit smoothies or juices.

Cooked fruit

Peel and core fruit before cooking.

Cut fruit into bite-sized pieces or slices.

Cook the fruit in various ways, such as baking, poaching, or grilling.

Serve cooked fruit with various sauces, such as custard, whipped cream, or ice cream.

Juiced fruit

Wash all fruit thoroughly before juicing.

The fruit should be free of any seeds or pits.

Juice fruit in a juicer or blender.

Serve juiced fruit immediately or store it in the refrigerator for later.

Here are some additional tips for preparing fruit:

Store fruit in a cool, dark place.

Eat fruit within a few days of purchase.

Avoid overripe fruit, as it may be mushy or taste sour.

Yogurt

Yogurt is an adaptable food that can be eaten any time of day due to its high protein and calcium content. It can also be utilized in a variety of dishes because it is a versatile component.

Here are some yogurt recipes and preparation tips:

Plain yogurt

Plain yogurt can be enjoyed independently or used as a base for smoothies, sauces, or dips.

Heat milk to 180 degrees Fahrenheit to make plain yogurt, then cool to 110 degrees Fahrenheit. Stir in 1 tablespoon of plain yogurt and allow it to sit warmly for 8-12 hours or until it has thickened.

Store plain yogurt in the refrigerator for up to 1 week.

Flavored yogurt

Flavored yogurt can be made by adding fresh fruit, honey, or granola to plain yogurt.

Combine 1 cup of plain yogurt with 1/2 cup of fresh fruit, one tablespoon of honey, or 1/2 cup of granola to make your flavored yogurt. Stir until well combined.

Store flavored yogurt in the refrigerator for up to 3 days.

Yogurt parfaits

Yogurt parfaits are a delicious and nutritious way to start your day. Layer yogurt, fruit, granola, and nuts in a glass or jar.

To make your yogurt parfait, combine 1/2 cup of yogurt with 1/4 cup of fruit, 1/4 cup of granola, and 1/4 cup of nuts.

Yogurt smoothies

Smoothies made with yogurt are an efficient and quick way to get daily fruits and veggies. Combine yogurt, fruit, milk, and ice until smooth.

To make your yogurt smoothie, combine 1 cup of yogurt, 1 cup of fruit, 1 cup of milk, and 1 cup of ice in a blender and blend until smooth.

Add other ingredients to your smoothie, such as honey, peanut butter, or protein powder.

Yogurt sauces

Yogurt sauces are a delicious and healthy way to flavor your food. They can be used as a dip for vegetables, a dressing for salads, or a sauce for chicken or fish.

Combine yogurt, lemon juice, olive oil, salt, and pepper to make your yogurt sauce. Whisk until well combined.

Add other ingredients to your yogurt sauce, such as garlic, herbs, or spices.

Yogurt dips

Yogurt dips are a delicious and healthy way to enjoy your favorite vegetables. They can be made with plain yogurt or flavored yogurt.

Combine yogurt, herbs, spices, and salt to dip your yogurt. Whisk until well combined.

Add other ingredients to your yogurt dip, such as garlic, lemon juice, or honey.

I hope these yogurt recipes and preparation tips help you find delicious and healthy ways to enjoy yogurt.

Trail Mix

Trail mix is a tasty and healthy snack that is great for eating on the go. It is also a great way to get daily fruits, nuts, and seeds.

Here is a simple trail mix recipe:

Ingredients:

1 cup nuts (almonds, cashews, peanuts, etc.)

1 cup dried fruit (raisins, cranberries, apricots, etc.)

1 cup seeds (chia, flax, pumpkin, etc.)

1/2 cup chocolate chips (optional)

Instructions:

Add all ingredients in a large bowl.

Refrigerate or store in an airtight container at room temperature for two weeks.

Here are some tips for making trail mix:

Be innovative with your ingredients. When it comes to trail mix, the possibilities are almost endless. You can use any nuts, dried fruit, or seeds you like.

Add other ingredients, such as granola, oats, or protein powder, to make your trail mix more nutritious.

If you are making trail mix for kids, you can omit the chocolate chips or use a healthier alternative, such as dried fruit or nuts.

Trail mix is a great snack to pack for school, work, or on a hike. It is also a healthy and delicious way to satisfy your sweet tooth.

Desserts

Desserts are sweet, typically high in sugar, fat, and calories, and are usually eaten at the end of a meal. They can be made from various ingredients, including fruits, nuts, chocolate, and sugar.

some popular desserts includes: Cake, Pie, Cookies, Ice cream, Brownies, Pudding, Trifle, Crème brûlée, Tiramisu, Soufflé

Desserts can be enjoyed independently or with other foods, such as coffee, tea, or fruit. They can also make other desserts, such as trifle or ice cream cake.

Here are some tips for making desserts:

Use high-quality ingredients. The value of your ingredients will make a big difference in the taste of your desserts.

Be precise with your measurements. It is important to be precise with your measurements when making desserts, as even a small difference can affect the outcome.

Follow the recipe carefully. Don't be tempted to change the recipe, which can affect the outcome.

Don't overbake your desserts. Overbaking can make them dry and crumbly.

Let your desserts cool completely before serving. This will help them to hold their shape and prevent them from falling apart.

Chocolate Brownies

Ingredients:

1 cup (2 sticks) unsalted butter, melted

1 cup unsweetened cocoa powder

1 cup sugar

1 cup packed light brown sugar

Four large eggs

Two teaspoons of vanilla extract

One teaspoon salt

1 cup all-purpose flour

1 cup semisweet chocolate chips

Instructions:

Preheat oven to (175 degrees C). Grease and flour in an 8x8-inch baking pan.

Whisk together the melted butter, cocoa powder, sugar, and brown sugar in a large bowl until smooth.

The salt and vanilla essence are added after beating each egg one at a time.

Beat in the flour a little at a time, just until incorporated. Add the chocolate chunks and stir.

Bake for 25 to 30 minutes, or until a toothpick inserted in the center comes out clean, after pouring the batter into the prepared pan.

Before cutting and serving, let the brownies cool fully.

Here are some tips for making chocolate brownies:

Use high-quality cocoa powder. The quality of your cocoa powder will make a big difference in the taste of your brownies.

Don't overmix the batter. Overmixing can make the brownies tough.

Don't overbake the brownies, as this can make them dry and crumbly.

Let the brownies cool completely before cutting and serving. This will help them to hold their shape and prevent them from falling apart.

Enjoy your brownies! Brownies are a delicious and decadent dessert that is perfect for any occasion.

Apple Pie

Ingredients:

For the crust:

1 1/2 cups all-purpose flour

One teaspoon sugar

1/2 teaspoon salt

1/4 cup (1/2 stick) unsalted butter, chilled and cut into small pieces

1/4 cup shortening, chilled and cut into small pieces

5 to 6 tablespoons of ice water

For the filling:

6 cups peeled, cored, and thinly sliced Granny Smith apples

1/2 cup sugar

1/4 cup all-purpose flour

One teaspoon of ground cinnamon

1/2 teaspoon ground nutmeg

1/4 teaspoon ground cloves

1/4 teaspoon salt

One tablespoon of lemon juice

1/4 cup (1/2 stick) unsalted butter, cut into small pieces

For the egg wash:

One large egg

One tablespoon water

Instructions:

Whisk the salt, flour, and sugar in a large bowl to make the crust. Add the butter and shortening and use your fingers to work the butter and shortening into the flour until it's coarse and crumbs.

Drizzle in the ice water, one tablespoon at a time, tossing with a fork until the dough comes together.

Refrigerate the dough for at least 30 mins after forming it into a disk and covering it with plastic wrap.

To make the filling, combine the apples, sugar, flour, cinnamon, nutmeg, cloves, salt, and lemon juice in a large bowl. Toss to coat.

Set the oven's temperature to 425 °F (220 °C).

The dough should be rolled out to a 12-inch circle on a lightly dusted surface.

Transfer the dough to a 9-inch pie plate and trim the edges. Pour the filling into the prepared pie crust.

Dot the top of the filling with the butter.

Whisk the egg and water together in a small bowl. Brush the egg wash over the top of the pie crust.

Bake the pie for 30 minutes, then reduce the heat to (190 degrees C) and bake for 30-35 mins until the crust is golden brown and the filling is bubbling.

Allow the pie to cool fully before serving.

Here are some tips for making apple pie:

Use a variety of apples for the filling.

Granny Smith apples are a good choice for their tartness, but you can add other apples, such as Honeycrisp, Fuji, or Gala.

Don't overcrowd the pie crust with the filling. The filling should come about 1 inch below the top of the crust.

Don't overbake the pie. Overbaking can make the crust tough and the filling dry. This will help the filling set and the crust to become flaky.

Enjoy your apple pie!

Ice Cream

Ingredients:

2 cups whole milk

1 cup heavy cream

1 cup sugar

One teaspoon of vanilla extract

Instructions:

The milk, cream, and sugar should all be combined in a medium pan.

Stirring occasionally, cook over medium heat until the sugar dissolves.

Add the vanilla extract after taking the pan off the heat.

As the manufacturer directs, pour the ingredients into an ice cream machine and churn.

Once the ice cream is churned, transfer it to an airtight container.

Finally, refrigerate it for at least 4 hours or overnight.

Serve and enjoy!

Tips for making ice cream:

Use high-quality ingredients. The quality of your ingredients will make a big difference in the taste of your ice cream.

Be precise with your measurements. When making ice cream, it is important to be precise with your measurements, as even a small difference can affect the outcome.

Don't overchurn your ice cream. Overchurning can make your ice cream icy.

Let your ice cream freeze for at least 4 hours or overnight. This will help it to set and become scoopable.

Enjoy your ice cream!

Other ice cream recipes you can try:

Chocolate ice cream: Substitute 1 cup of unsweetened cocoa powder for 1 cup of milk.

Strawberry ice cream: Add 1 cup of fresh strawberries to the mixture before churning.

Mint chocolate chip ice cream: Add 1/2 cup of chopped mint chocolate chips to the ice cream mixture before churning.

Peanut butter cup ice cream: Add 1/2 cup of peanut butter cups to the ice cream mixture before churning.

Cookies and cream ice cream: Add 1/2 cup of cookies to the ice cream mixture before churning.

Be creative and have fun with your ice cream recipes!

Conclusion

In conclusion, this cookbook has provided various easy and delicious recipes perfect for people with chronic fatigue syndrome. The recipes are all low-fat, low-sugar, and gluten-free, filled with nutrients that can help improve your energy levels and overall health.

I hope this cookbook inspired you to cook healthier, more delicious meals. Remember, eating a healthy diet is one part of managing chronic fatigue syndrome.

Please talk to your doctor if you struggle to manage your

Thank you for reading this cookbook! I hope that you enjoy the recipes.